I0410693

January, 1987

I felt the lump
    as I showered.

In that moment
    the expectation
    of having fun
    at a birthday party

    diminished.

BREAST CANCER, AN EMOTIONAL JOURNEY (30 YEARS LATER)

MARGARET PHALOR BARNHART
Christian Author and Inspirational Speaker

Text and Illustrations by Margaret Barnhart

Self published in 2016. Book can be purchased on Amazon and retail book sellers around the world. It is available on Kindle as well as all e-books. Kindle has an app that will work on most tablets.

Paperback Book ISBN: 978-1537555041
E-Book ISBN: 1537555049

Table of Contents

Acknowledgement

Roger Reinardy and I have never met. Over thirty years ago, when I was on a six-month course of chemotherapy, it was his needlepoint design called "Penguin Promenade" that occupied 52 hours of my time. My eyes were weak, and I had difficulty reading. However, this needlework used larger holes with various colors of yarn.

I started in the upper right corner and worked my way to the left. As the black penguins moved toward the rainbow, my mood lightened and lifted me out of depression. Roger's design was just what I needed. Recently, I was able to track him down in Minnesota and received his permission to use a rendition of his design on the cover of "Journey Unknown."

He wrote back to me, "Marge, you do me honor by taking this piece to a whole new level. Of course, you have my permission to use it on the cover of your book. My late wife was the business part of the company, and I was the design end. She would have been very happy to see our design in "Breast Cancer, an Emotional Journey."

Thank you, dear Roger

Note From the Author

Life's journey sent me on a search for identity and control. As a child, a daughter, and a sister, I explored and challenged. The years of education included advanced degrees in Elementary Education (Capital University, Columbus, Ohio), Guidance and Counseling (Miami University, Oxford, Ohio), and Art Therapy (Wright State University, Dayton, Ohio).

The 28 years of my first marriage included mothering two sons, many household moves to accommodate my husband's job desires, full time work for 17 years in a number of Ohio school systems, and extensive travel.

Chaos resulted when my contract as a school counselor was non-renewed. Prior to this time (16 years) I never had a negative evaluation. Now my principal said I didn't smile enough, children didn't run up to me for hugs, and I needed to schedule more classroom guidance classes. Trying to please my evaluator, I worked to fit my being into the mold he wanted and thought I could do it. I ate lunch while working with children, and I managed one trip to the bathroom each day. Time for individual counseling was reduced. I took work home and made parent phone calls in the evening.

In the process of trying to satisfy my principal, I lost myself. My self-esteem shattered and I became depressed. Between the vote of the school board in March and the last day of school in June, I lost ten pounds and felt the loss of a hundred relationships with children, their parents, and the teachers. At this job I had two buildings with a principal in each. My second principal wrote a glowing letter of recommendation!

After signing up for unemployment I took time to recuperate and did not have the emotional strength to go for interviews in other school districts. I decided to attend graduate school and signed up for five classes, all in different programs. Art therapy was interesting and I chose to go the direction.

By taking classes for two summers and one school year, I earned a master's degree. I interviewed for and was offered a job in a school district about 25 miles from home. I was required to travel between two elementary schools and all was well until the day I felt the lump in my breast in March of 1987.

Once the diagnosis was made, I was scheduled for a mastectomy. Two weeks later my internist called me in and talked about the need for chemotherapy. Suddenly, the accumulation of wisdom and experience was inadequate. My religious beliefs flew away. I felt lost.

In May I returned to my schools for two weeks so I could prepare 5th grade students transferring to middle school. During the next school year I returned to my schools, even though I was still receiving chemotherapy. I thought as the treatments came to an end, I wouldn't have as many side effects. That wasn't true. To begin, the 25 mile drive wore me out before I arrived at work.

My main building had three floors and my office was at the top. I quickly became physically and mentally exhausted. The principal and I agreed that I would stay home on Wednesdays for as long as necessary.

I started working full time again in 1988, but quickly deteriorated. The first week of October

I admitted that I didn't have the strength to go on. I was approved for disability retirement at the age of 48.

Coming back from the brink of despair, I look to the future with the light of God on my shoulder. Looking in the mirror conveys my submission to a spiritual identity and fully accepting me as a child of God. This is the peace that passes all understanding.

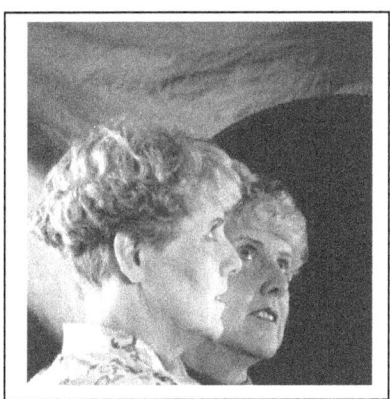

Photo by Jim Witmer 1987

Since that time in the 1980's my life changed considerably from not working, to trying to rebuild my body after chemotherapy, especially seeking to strengthen my legs. After a year with no improvement, a new exercise trainer had me lie on my back and push up 10# weighted disks. I felt something shift and eventually learned that my coccyx had been damaged.

Breast Cancer, an Emotional Journey

After a year and a half of intense pain (especially when sitting) I accepted the suggestion of my breast surgeon that he could remove the coccyx and it was 50/50 if that would help. I was desperate for relief and had the surgery.

Ultimately I learned that the surgeon not only removed my coccyx, but also cut the tendons and ligaments that support the pelvic floor, leaving me with pelvic instability. It is still a problem today.

I feel sad that my 28 year marriage ended in divorce. My husband gave me two sons, whom I love dearly, financial security, and many travel opportunities.

I spent many years wanting to live in southern Arizona, a place I had visited numerous times. It fulfilled a need I couldn't find in Ohio. The cloudy days and weather in general was a big factor in my long term depression.

Charles Barnhart and I married and moved into a lovely home in Troy, Ohio. Within that first year we joined a group travelling to the Holy Land.

I had an eye opening experience on the way home. We had a four hour layover in Rome. While

reclining on a bench to rest my "sitter," I became aware of pain developing throughout my body and my sinus cavities swelling.

That was the beginning of the move to Green Valley, in Southern Arizona. Several years passed before we were able to complete the move but living here has made all the difference in my health. Most days are sunny, the air is clear, and the mountains are nearby.

ooooooooooooooooooooooooooooooooo

My breast cancer was diagnosed and treated in the year 1987. The writings and art in this book are from that year. My doctor, after reading some of the poetry told me to self-publish which I did in a book titled, "Journey Unknown." It is no longer in print.

[Thirty years cancer free.]

I decided to tell my story once more because women (and sometimes men) are still having mastectomies and chemotherapy, and various forms of radiation. Their lives are filled with emotions of all sorts. Reading this book will help them, and you, find support and an understanding that they are not alone.

Tributes

"Margaret Phalor Barnhart's "Breast Cancer, an Emotional Journey" is an honest look at how she dealt with her journey through uncharted territory for her—breast cancer. The physical treatments are well known and provide a standard of care meant to heal. However, the emotional aspects of dealing with a cancer diagnosis are powerful and terrifying.

I highly recommend this book for each individual, but they should know that many, such as this author, have triumphantly completed the same journey."

Editorial Review for Amazon Kindle
By John McClure

Breast Cancer, an Emotional Journey

"Sometimes when we experience pain, it is merely God's way of stretching out spaces in our hearts for the joy that follows. Experiencing cancer is a painful process, both physically and emotionally.

"Breast Cancer, an Emotional Journey," filled my heart with joy and made me know that life's journey has been paved and made ready by God. Margaret Barnhart's brilliance, through poetry, has helped to make each day's journey more joyful for me."

Zora Kramer Brown, Washington, D.C.
Founder Breast Cancer Resource Committee

oooooooooooooooooooooooo

"[This] book is a marvelous gift. It will be a resource to pastors and anyone who seeks to comfort and help those who are battling cancer. It will be a source of strength for anyone who undergoes surgery and treatment for cancer. I have found it to be a healing gift in my own life, and I recommend it highly."

Kenneth H. Sauer,
Former Bishop Southern Ohio Synod,
Evangelical Lutheran Church in America

I received the book, and the day I got it, I sat down and read it cover to cover, including all the reviews, intros, etc. I seldom do that … I related to all the poems and articles, even though I didn't always have exactly the same feelings. She certainly has a gift of expression …"

Jo Anne

oooooooooooooooooooooO

"Breast Cancer, an Emotional Journey," is authentic, chilling, desperate, and encouraging. You are an amazing woman; you truly live a victorious life!"

LaVerne

oooooooooooooooooooooO

"A poignant expression of feelings and emotions, paints a picture of the breast cancer experience that can be visualized and felt by all.

Susan Leigh, Oncology Nurse

Breast Cancer, an Emotional Journey

"...an excellent source of support for many breast cancer patients. Her words and expressions related to her journey through her episode of breast cancer are expressed with great feeling and understanding. Meaningful and touching."

Sidney F. Miller, MD
Director, The Ohio State University Burn Care, Columbus, Ohio

"I love Margaret's book. My only regret is that my sister died of breast cancer before having a chance to read it. I am giving it to her daughter."

Bobbi

ooooooooooooooooooooo

"In April, 2016, Encanterra Writing Club (near Phoenix) was very fortunate to discover Margaret. We wanted to find an author who would share his/her writing with us. She was a perfect fit and when the Book Club and Bible Study groups heard she was coming, they wanted to be included.

"The audience had different interests, but she kept all engrossed. She read portions of her cancer story which is so well written they inspire, inform and give hope."

Nel Adcock

PREFACE

Statistics can be manipulated to convey whatever message the writer chooses. They can be used to frighten, to impress, to inspire, or to prove a point. In the year 1987, I was the "one" out of the statistical eleven. There has been no recurrence.

For 46 years I was healthy and energetic, never able to appreciate the struggle of many who endure constant pain and illness. For almost two years, I was a patient in physical discomfort and emotional turmoil. I was dependent on the medical community. I was scared.

The writings and artwork contained in this book were initiated as my own therapy. When thoughts tumbled compulsively within my mind, especially at night, I sought relief through pencil and paper.

I was coping with many degrees of loss, and each aspect of the illness—mastectomy, cancer, and chemotherapy—started me through the grief cycle of shock, denial, anger, bargaining, depression, and acceptance.

Because these cycles were intermingled and overlapping, I often felt that I was the ball in a game of handball, never knowing which wall I would bounce from next.

"Loss" seems to be the primary issue. Loss occurs in many realms, and in order to remain psychologically healthy, every person must come to terms with their losses and find resolution.

Encouraged by my doctor to share my experiences with others, I discovered the power contained herein. Some cried. Many expressed having feelings similar to mine but from other causes.

Sharing my story at such an intensely personal level was frightening. Following my first group presentation, I imaged myself as an old-fashioned camera, opened at the back, with the film exposed. I hoped I hadn't been damaged.

You, the reader, are invited to walk the path I traveled 30 years ago. If my journey becomes overwhelming, pause and reflect your thoughts and emotions through any creative means. I am convinced that the insight you gain will be well worth the effort.

For surely I know the
plans I have for you,
says the Lord,

plans for your welfare
and not for harm,

to give you a future
with hope.

Jeremiah 29:11
(NRSV)

ELEVATOR

A lump is an intruder in one's body. It triggers an overwhelming amount of emotion. I had been through this experience one other time, three years prior. I adamantly refused to sign consent for mastectomy, and it was not needed. (The doctor said the biopsy showed something that was a word too big and complicated for me to understand!) I was so innocent.

In January of 1987, I discovered a new lump in my breast. An antibiotic was prescribed, but after two weeks, there was no change. I was referred to a surgeon who determined that this lump was a benign cyst.

More intense examination led to the discovery of another lump that was biopsied. Because of its location near the sternum, it had not shown on my last mammogram.

My small town surgeon told me if there was cancerous material found, the breast would be removed. I asked about a lumpectomy. His response was that mastectomies have been done since the 1800's and are the best treatment.

Now I had another problem. I wasn't happy with such a rigid position and told him I wanted a second opinion. He replied that he didn't know why. I was now even more convinced that I needed another perspective.

Traveling to a larger town, I received a second opinion confirming my surgeon's recommendation. The explanation was quite different. The size of the lump, the size of my breast, and the lump's proximity to my chest wall indicated clearly that I needed a modified radical mastectomy. The decision would be made while I remained under anesthesia.

The "elevator dream" occurred three days after the biopsy of tissue removed from my breast, was labeled "suspicious."

This dream was a powerful indicator of what was ahead. The combined sense of fear and hope was poignant. This was a recurring sensation throughout my journey.

Discovery

January

I felt the lump
    as I showered.
In that moment
    the expectation of having fun
    at a birthday party
    diminished.

Three years ago a cyst was
surgically removed. Here I go
again.

Should I call the doctor Monday?
Surely I'm over reacting. Wait
several weeks. It may go away.

Socializing at the
celebration was hampered
by
    three trips to the
    bathroom to feel the lump
    that was still there.

Elevator Dream
February

It was a dark night.
A tall city building
      unfinished, under construction.
Seven stories completed.
Above them open girders.

Upon entering the elevator
I touch the button labeled "TOP."

Alone, I cling to the centerpole
as surrounding buildings diminish
and city lights dim.

This upward journey
leading to the unknown
creates PANIC . . .
TERROR!

Yet, an inner peace.

A strong sense
that the elevator is
connected to a cable that
I cannot see but know is
anchored.

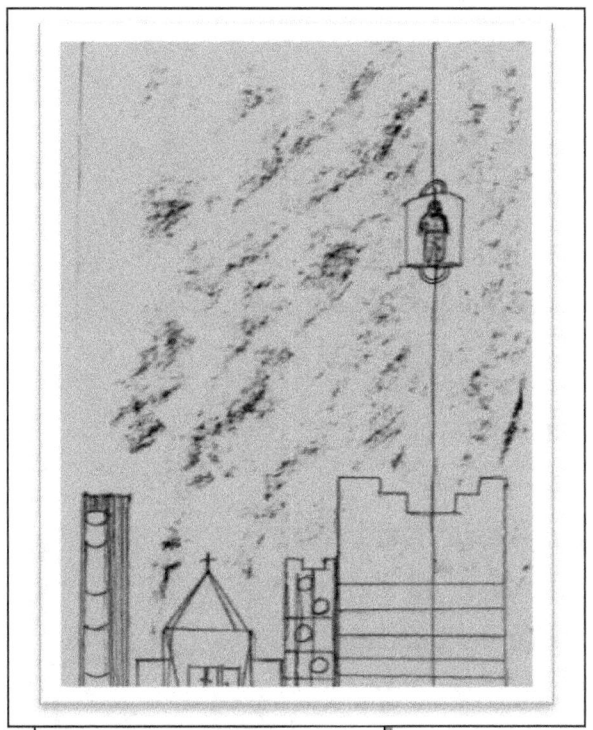

Elevator Dream

Timely Concerns
March

24 hours before:
—hospital pre-admission,
—radical mastectomy consent form signed,
—don't pack, but arrange items needed for
      personal care.

12 hours before:
—love me, my dear, and
      hold me tight;
—touch me and kiss me.

12 hours after:
—Yes, I know.
—Family surround me,
      suspend me,
—share my burden.

Breast Cancer, an Emotional Journey

24 hours after:
—nurses hovering
—feeling helpless
—searching the future.

36 hours after:
—thick gauze simulates my missing breast
—mental rehearsal of touching the lump.

48 hours after:
—doctor removing dressing;
—look; see; don't think.
—Begin to grieve this loss.

60 hours after:
—frustrated with eating left-handed;
—lonely; missing freedom;
—questioning others' reactions;
—rebelling; choosing hospital gown over
          satin and frills.

72 hours after:

My right breast is not me, and
yet I cry.

But I still have the other one;

I still have an arm and hand;

I am still alive!

The Breakfast Tray

March

"The doctor is coming," announces the
nurse,
—coming to remove the bandages."

"Here is your breakfast," smiles an aide,
—and swiftly goes her way.
My one-handed efforts to unseal the
juice go unrewarded.
The clank of the cart carrying
scissors and gauze;
The thought of cold eggs; the thought
of swallowing;

Emotions reeling,
Eyes focus on the breakfast tray,
Anger.

With absolute rage, I give myself permission.
Go ahead. Push that tray away.
Send it clear across the room.

Restraint. (smile) "Hello, Doctor!"

Going Home
March

Five days of hospital routine;
    —physical healing.

I've been patted and prodded, pampered,
    poked, and persuaded.
Tubes have been jerked,
    staples snipped.

I came focused on a lump.
I leave focused on a gap;
    —and statistics
    —and percentages
    —and fear of recurrence.
Going home means
    —looking in the closet
    —viewing myself through the
        eyes of others
Leaving the cocoon.

[1987 insurance covered me for 5 days in hospital.]

DAFFODILS

Anticipating the journey home produced an unexpected fear. Although I was healing physically, I wasn't sure I could face family and friends outside the hospital setting. I had adapted well to the hospital routine.

Going home meant a return to a life I had known before the diagnosis of cancer and the removal of my right breast. I had changed radically in six days' time. The intensity of my emotions frightened me, yet I buried them inside.

Daffodils took on far greater significance than they deserved. It so happened that I was in the hospital at the time of the American Cancer Society sale of daffodils as a fund raiser. Someone had purchased them for me.

My strong feelings about carrying the daffodils the day I left the hospital intrigue me

still. I had many options; yet, stoically, I held them while, at the same time, considering them a symbol that I hated.

Many months later, I met the nurse who had delivered the flowers, and she recalled her uncomfortable feelings. It made us both aware of how sensitive a person may be to this diagnosis of cancer.

Six weeks later I received daffodils in celebration of Easter. I placed them in a nice glass vase. By drawing them I was able to resolve the negative thoughts stirred earlier.

The friend who received my drawing on a note card later commented on the fact that I asked for it back. He was able to appreciate its importance to me.

I had never been on the receiving end of so much attention. The number of cards that came surprised me, and I was impressed with the careful selection of the messages. I wondered if anyone else ever experienced the negative feelings that were aroused in me.

The Yellow Daffodils
March

I didn't want the daffodils
—a gift from an unknown donor!
I took them only to be polite.

Daffodils are supposed to be a cheerful
ray, a yellow, delicate creation.

I wanted to deny them a place in my
hands as I left the hospital that day.

Why hadn't I given them to the old
man in the room next to mine?
Why was I taking them home?
Why didn't I ask my husband to carry them?

The daffodils loomed large as I sat in the
wheelchair being pushed through the
corridor. I considered dropping them in a
wastebasket.

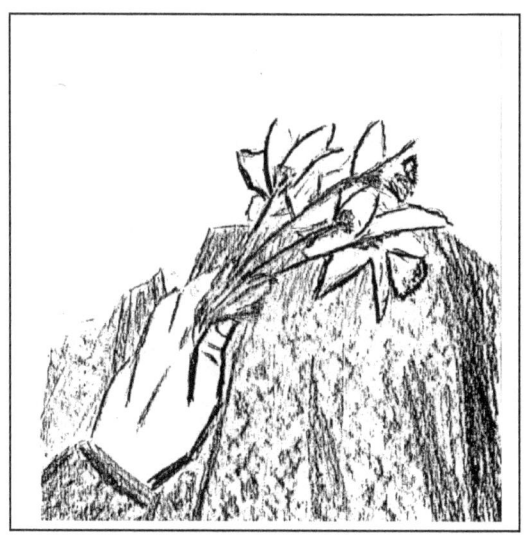

Surely, they were the label
that conveyed the message
that I had cancer.

My anger told me to slam them to the
floor to be crushed under the wheels!

At home they sat in a vase.
I hated looking at them
and was glad when they died.

Plants, Flowers and Cards
March

Plants, flowers, and cards
are bringing out the anger in me.
I don't want all these reminders of
my condition.
I don't want my condition.

[Mail delivery]

MORE CARDS

Plants, flowers, and cards help
me know *I am not alone.*
I suffer; I'm in pain;

But *enveloped by a cloud of love,*

I recover.

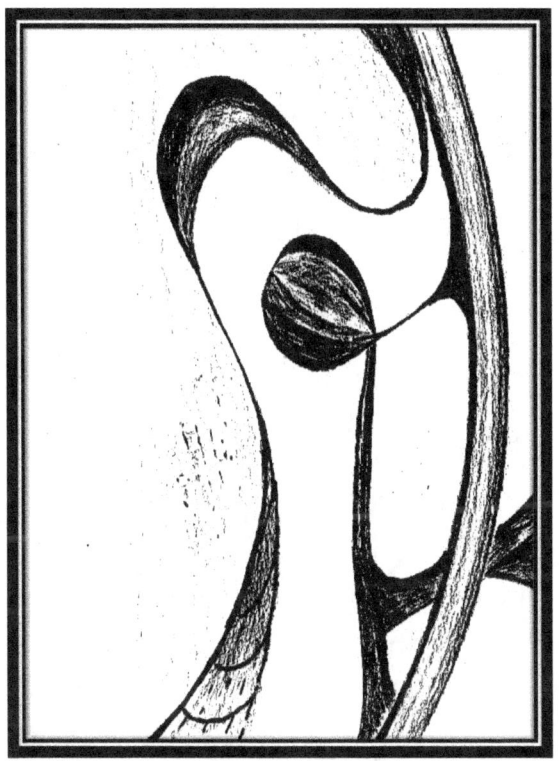

Half a Pound of Tissue

March

Half a pound of tissue and a lump the size of a
pea;   a malignant lump.   Cancer.

Half a pound of tissue scooped out of its shell;
        my breast.
        Nipple gone, skin folded over,
        stapled, muscles repositioned.

Look at the prosetheses,
        almost like normal. Sure!

Half a pound of tissue that nourished my sons
        as many years ago
        the nipple they sucked.

Half a pound of tissue never again
        to be touched or caressed.
Grief over half a pound of tissue?
        You bet.

Drawing for a Friend
April

A daffodil drawing for you, my friend;

An Easter celebration card for you as you wait
behind prison walls.

One for you, one for me, is my intent.
A way for me to celebrate life anew.

The daffodils of six weeks ago represented
cancer and fear.
The daffodils of today, a resurgence, a rebirth.

Friend in prison,

I think so often of the bars that limit you
physically, but not spiritually, and recognize the
thoughts and fears that imprison me.

The drawing I send to you, my friend, will be the
only one made, for my energy is spent.
Enjoy the card, my friend, and, when your need
is satisfied, would you be so kind to return it to
me?

A friend understands the request.

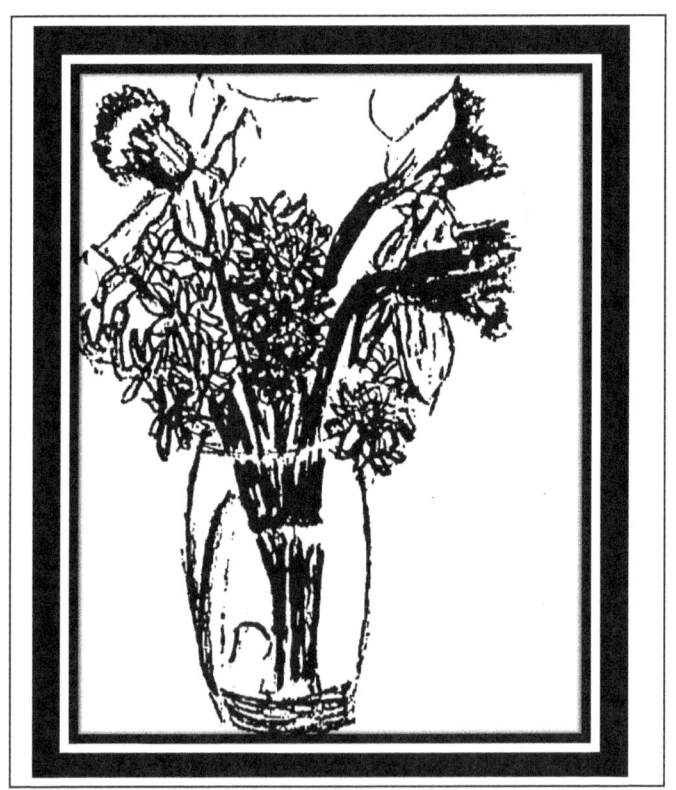

TURBULENCE

My decision to accept the doctor's recommendation for six months of chemotherapy sent me into a world of fear. It was unlike any I had ever experienced.

My father died of Lymphoma at the age of 71. The last time I saw him was at the hospital with bags of chemicals dripping into his veins. I was surprised when my mother told me that my dad had been diagnosed with Hodgkin's Disease when he was in his 40's. He had been treated with radiation and lived 29 more years. That was encouraging.

Even so, it was very difficult for me to accept the introduction of drugs into my body. Along with the powerful drugs was a medication intended to prevent nausea, and for me, it worked effectively throughout the six-month period. That surprised many people.

Side effects took their toll on me. The journey of the unknown led me on a turbulent path. Although I was able to work part time and maintain some other activities, there were many "down" days where I did little other than sit and sometimes work on stitchery.

A feeling that I had lost control pervaded my thoughts, and I examined the meaning of the word "control" repeatedly. My emotional state was in turmoil, with many lows and few, if any, highs.

My doctor suggested I view chemotherapy as a preventive measure, like the insect spray used in a bed of flowers. That imagery helped. The loving support of many people carried me through this period.

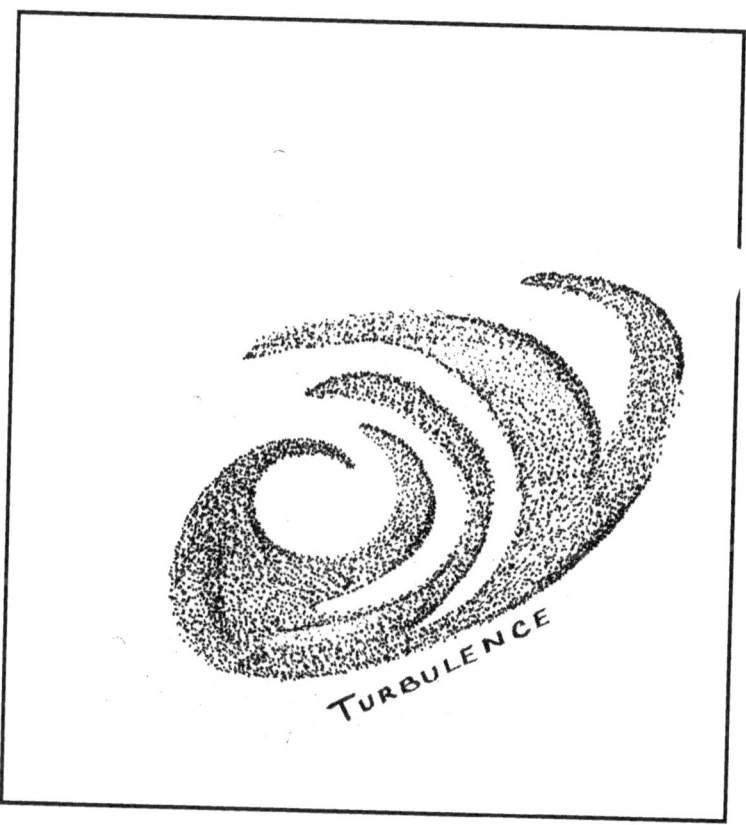

The Chemotherapy Crisis

April

"Good news," said the surgeon.
"Lymph nodes are clear, we
got it all."

"Not so good," says the internist, as
   two weeks after surgery he
    explains that for my type cancer I
   need at least six months
   of chemical intervention.

But I hate to experience nausea,
   and I don't want to lose my hair.

My father endured the treatment
   for a year before he died.
   I fear the chemicals.
   Do I also fear the possibility of dying?

Fear and Tears

April

Listen to me, doctor, understand
my tears.

The pain of losing a breast has
dimmed.

Fear of chemotherapy
and unknown side effects immobilizes me.

Pills to take and the first IV,
halfway through the night

    I sit,
    afraid to fall asleep.

I want to stay awake,

so I know I am alive.

A Hand Full of Hair
April

Three weeks of chemotherapy.
What a drag.
I need to get out—do something fun.

"Let's go to the ice show tonight,"
suggests my husband.
Ideal.
A deal.

A shower and a quick shampoo,
A hand full of hair!
A wad of hair!

Stunning disbelief

    and simultaneous knowledge
    that I am not to be spared
    this side effect.

Ice show, yes. Fun, no.

At least in the darkness,
The audience cannot see
The flow of tears cascading.

Loss of Hair

April

Is it vanity that makes me cry
as my hair comes out by the handful three
weeks after the first IV?

Or is it one more bout
with the reality of cancer?
Somehow, baldness does not fit
my image of femininity.

Shopping for a wig is pure drudgery.

Yes, I know.

The person is more than the body

I know, This, too, shall pass.
But for now, the pain is very real.

Drawing Myself

May

On this day, looking into a mirror,
I drew myself.

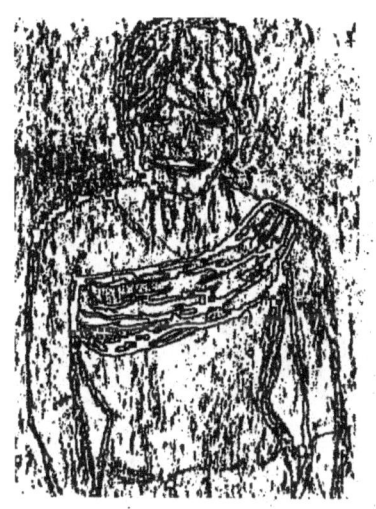

The tactile stimulation
in the use of charcoal
aided the process of acceptance.

Shopping for a Breast

May

What is the proper attitude
one assumes
when shopping for a breast?

Naming it a prosthesis
may be more dignified,
 but, in my mind the two do not
equate.

Just walk right up and say,
        "I need a ... a ... a ..."

Does one confront this task
        —seriously? —jokingly?   —alone?

Remember when I
        —hid behind towels?
        —coughed in church to
         avoided saying "Jesus' breast?"
        —ordered chicken legs when I
        really wanted   a . . . a . . . ?

Three Reflections
May

I look in the mirror. Who am I?
In the reflection I see
      a curly-headed blond.

Out into the world I go,
feeling the wig
around my head,
wondering who notices,
      feigning confidence,
        trying to forget.

I look in the mirror. Who am I now?
In the reflection I see
a thin-haired old woman.

Into my world of pain I hide, aware of
the hair loss, telling others it's like a
      baby's fine hair,

trying to deny the real thoughts,
    the old woman thoughts.

I look in the mirror. Who am I now?
In the reflection,
    I see a cover-up.

Feeling my head getting cold
   in the comfort of my home,
   I add a scarf,
      that offers warmth;
      that hides reality.

A scarf. And yet, another symbol that

    I have CANCER

Control

May

I've lost control.
I flounder. Yet,
I sense an inward flow
from a spiritual source that goes
through me and radiates out to
others--

      deepening in meaning as it travels,

      continuing in its movement back to me

      and giving meaning to my life.

But—what do I control?

Unexpected happenings cause change

      . . . physical

      . . . emotional

      . . . mental

      . . . spiritual

      . . . social.

What controls me?

Spiritual Insights
May

Yellow is all around me
               and within me.

Yellow is spiritual.

Yellow brings peace.

Living for Today

May

I've quit fighting
—because I've given up? given in? NO!

It is more like giving over, giving way.
Too much is outside my control.

I'll accept what is.
I'll live for today.

I cannot add one day to my life.
I'll do what I can for the moment.
I'll walk through the rainbow and
        add color wherever I can.

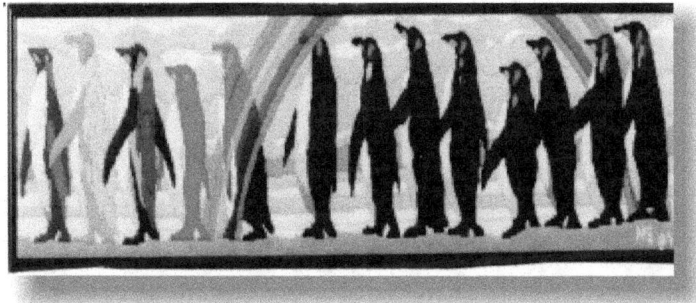

"Penguin Promenade" designed by Roger W. Reinardy
Horizons Designs, Inc. Used by permission.

Halfway Through

July

Three months of chemo completed.

Halfway through,

> a relief, a sense of satisfaction.

Side effects a nuisance

- ➤ exhausted but hyper

- ➤ fingers numb

- ➤ overstimulated by noise and light
- ➤ metallic taste like aluminum foil
        explosion with spices
- ➤ weakened vision
- ➤ poor concentration
- ➤ thermostat wildly fluctuating.

However, little nausea and hair loss abating.
I've come this far.

Facing the next IV--depression
A fear that it may never end.

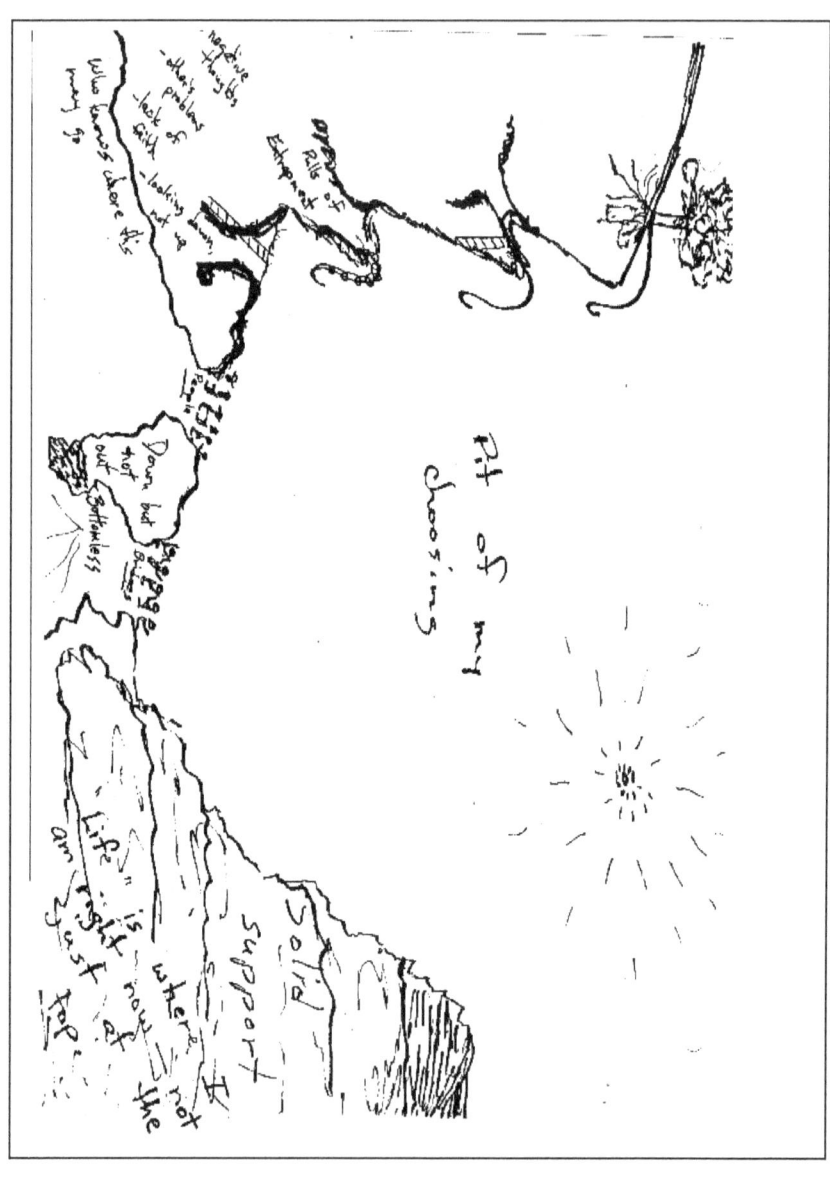

Is it Cancer?

July

A cough, a sneeze.
Is it normal? Or, is it
    a side effect of chemotherapy?
Or, is it
    CANCER?

A headache
    different from others.
Is it sinus? Or, is it
    a side effect of chemotherapy?
Or, is it
    CANCER?

A skin mole
    not of importance before the diag-
    nosis of breast cancer.

Now it looks suspicious; yet,
           too petty to mention.

Still a worry.

Is it CANCER?

Will I think this way the rest of my life?

           Or, after chemotherapy ends,
                   will I relax?

The unanswered question still remains—

Did I have cancer?

           Or

Do I have CANCER?

Chemotherapy Miseries

August

The TASTE

    . . . salt and spices explode within

    . . . eat this, eat that

    . . . seeking resolution.

The SOUND
noises amplified

    —loading the dishwasher

    —breaking ice cubes out of trays

    —stirring sugar in the tea

    —slamming a cupboard door

    a multitude of kitchen sounds.

The TOUCH
numbness resulting in

    —objects dropped

    —burning myself

The VISION
     . . . looking out through inner fog
     . . . lights at night florescent
     . . . reading—a chore demanding
    too much energy to concentrate.

The occasional HALLUCINATION of
GIGANTIC
       . . . I mean elephantine!
—fat tongue licking fat lips
—eyelids stretching over enlarged eyeballs
—huge fingers reaching out from puffy hands.

The SPEECH
. . . slowed, slurred
. . . searching for words
. . . struggling to organize thoughts.

The MUSCLES
. . . that tighten and cramp at the site
    of my mastectomy

The BODY TEMPERATURE
. . . cold
      —shivering cold,
. . . then hot
      —HOT!
Volcanic style.

And the TIREDNESS
. . . I can't lie down hard enough!

The Sixth Month
August

The end is in sight.

Five months behind me, one ahead. Yet, each time
I say "the end," I fear.

I fear the possibility—
     the possibility of cancer cells
     that I never knew were there,
     multiplying in my body,
     unaffected by drugs.

I fear the possibility—
     the possibility of a need
     for more chemotherapy.

I fear death by cancer—
the possibility,
a possibility I didn't consider earlier.

How can I feel excited or relieved about a last round when there are no guarantees that this will always be the last round?

Waiting for a Diagnosis

September

Yesterday, I thought I was dying

  —dying of brain cancer
  as I awaited the results of a CT scan
  because of headaches that
  for two months now come and go.

I know someone who just died of brain cancer.
Awaiting a diagnosis can seem an eternity.

Do I plan for next week, next month?
  --or is the future cancelled?
  —or at least postponed?

Do I fear death, or do I fear losing life?
  —or the quality of life
  to which I am accustomed?

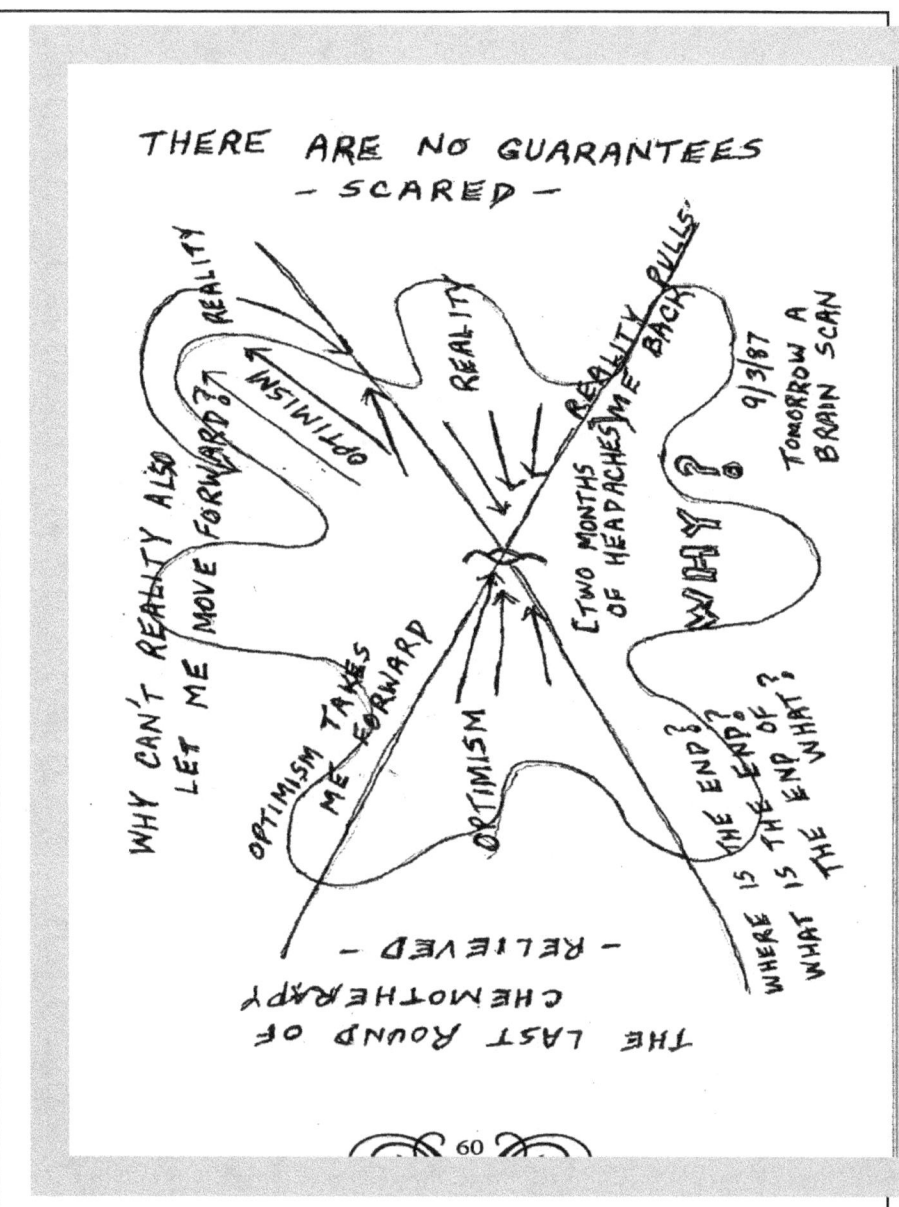

Today, the phone call came.

Scan normal,

    —cause of headaches, unknown.

Headaches now seem unimportant.

Cancer cells are not the cause.

Will this fear of cancer remain forever?

    ---a curse

    I relentlessly bear?

RAINBOW

Acceptance and resolution have involved a spiritual element I've had difficulty defining. For years I've been examining my faith and redefining my relationship with God. The artwork I relied on when at a loss for words tended to clarify the sense of connectedness.

The theme occurred repeatedly beginning with the cable in the "Elevator Dream" and continuing in the burst of light in "Pit of my Choosing," and radiating with the penguins in their walk through the rainbow.

Our journeys are different but have commonalities. Many refer to God and ask him the "BIG" questions. The "Why" and the "Where is He?"

I tried to just live in the moment. I did not choose cancer and many of the days when I was under the influence of chemotherapy drugs, I questioned if I was capable of controlling my thoughts and emotions.

One of the most stressful days was when I had one pill left to take. My internal thoughts kept ranting, "Don't take this last pill. It might be the one that kills you." On the other side of my brain I heard, "This last pill might be the one that saves your life and prevents you from having a recurrence."

I finally took the pill.

Since I have been cancer free for 30 years it was probably the right choice!

Push or Take it Easy?

September

The six months of chemo have ended.

I have returned to work.

Work is 25 miles from my home.
Work is in two elementary buildings
        where I am a school counselor.

My office is on the third floor.
My legs are weak.

Life has not returned to a prior normal.
I have such limited energy.

Do I push to keep going?

How do I take it easy as some advise?

How long do co-workers and supervisors
        accept my limitations?

Becoming

September

In the past I've been heard to say,

"Stitchery and needlework are not my
line, wait until I'm old and have more
time." With chemo, I have the time.

Time to sit with a body that can't keep going and
        a mind that won't stop going
        and a need for a sense of control.

In and out the holes,
        needle and yarn, follow the pattern.
This I can control.

Penguins walking through a rainbow—
        black and white, becoming color. Changing.

I, too, am changing.
I can never be the same.

See page 63 and imagine the colors!

Acceptance of Loss of a Breast

September

When awakening from surgery six months ago,
    the pressing thought and immediate
    question centered on the loss of my breast.

"Is it gone?"

Acceptance has come in stages
 overshadowed and
 submerged by chemotherapy.

Acceptance has come in
    stages

     —when the doctor removed the bandages
     —when I looked . . . touched
     —when another looks . . . touches
     —when hugged.

Acceptance includes

> ➢ looking in the mirror,
> ➢ sensing the numbness,
> ➢ wearing a prosthesis,
> ➢ standing tall, and most of all,
> ➢ accepting me.

Accepting Life

September

Two weeks before surgery
        and the discovery of cancer,
I told a friend I figured I had lived half my
        life at the age of 46.

Yet, in the past six months,
I've mentally and emotionally
been preparing to die
        —when I had nosebleeds,
        —when I coughed with bronchitis,
        —when the headaches were severe,
convinced that cancer was consuming me.

In this last week of chemotherapy,
my focus has been on the word
"last"
        —wanting guarantees.

Acceptance relies on reality.

Six months ago, with a laugh,
my son predicted I would get hit by a car
on the way to the doctor for my last IV.

My son was wrong.

The Paradox

September

Cancer is a life-threatening disease.
People die of cancer—
>>>> many women,
>>>> many men.

Having cancer
>>>> does **not** mean
>>>> I
>>>> will die of cancer.

Cancer forced me to understand and accept that
my death will occur. When and how I do not
know. However, I feel stronger now about life
and live each day to the fullest.

How Am I?

October

This morning I realized that
  at a meeting I attended last night,
  not one person said, "How are you?"

For eight months, I have struggled
  with an answer to that question
  because, for eight months, I haven't
  known how I am.

I called my doctor and asked,

  "How am I?"

"You're not sick anymore!" he replied.

His response freed me—

  freed me to be well.

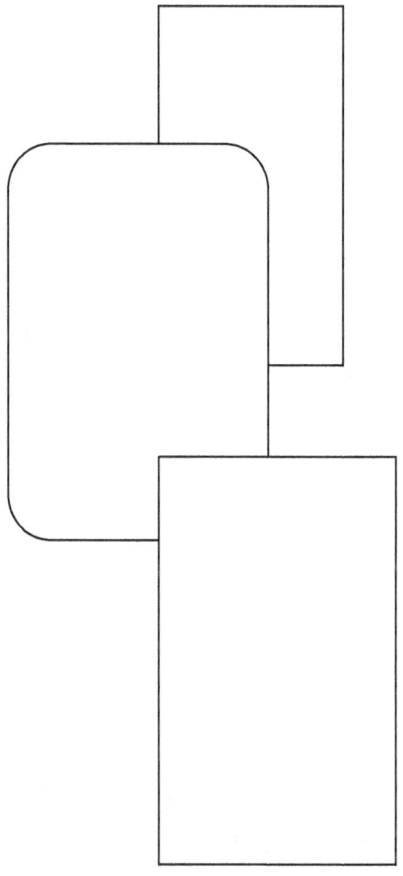

EPILOGUE

1988

Following my surgery and chemotherapy, I realized that all the focus had been on me. I was curious what others thought about my bout with cancer, and I sent a letter to family and close friends. You also may be interested in how things look from the other side.

February 23, 1988

Dear _____,

"It has been almost a year since I went into   the hospital, had the mastectomy, and heard the diagnosis of breast cancer. Three weeks later, I began chemotherapy treatments that lasted for six months.

What was your reaction when you first heard the news? What thoughts led to what actions or inactions? How did you view me as I dealt with the various aspects over a long period of time?

How has my experience related to your life?

Your response may be any length, any style, writing, or art work. When I publish, I'll use only your relationship to me. Your love and support have been of tremendous importance to me as I've struggled with the events of the past year."

From my husband of 26 years:

'My reaction upon first hearing the news was stunned and concerned about how you would react upon awakening from surgery. Then I wondered what effect this would have on our lives. I didn't give any thought to death, which surprises me. I was wondering how I could be supportive and do what was needed to facilitate recovery.

I tried to be more helpful, maybe a little beyond what I normally would do. I wanted to be more caring and concerned about you rather than myself. During chemo I again felt helpless and did what I could see to do. Adjustments were made, but I don't think any were dramatic."

From my two sons:

One lived out of town and the other was a senior in high school. They were at a loss as far as words go. Since I wasn't talking about it, neither did they.

From my mother:

"In mid-February, I fell and broke my leg. I had to use a walker and could not leave the house. You came to visit me and told me that you were going into the hospital to have breast surgery. You let me feel the tumor and told me what might happen. I was worried.

Your father had Hodgkin's Disease (a form of lymph cancer) in his 40's and was given six months to live. With many prayers and x-ray therapy, he was in remission until he reached 70.

I had been warned by the doctor that it could occur again, and this time the cancer started in the groin. Again, lymph cancer.

Naturally, when you told me about your impending surgery, I was really frightened. I could not be with you that day because of my broken leg.

Your sister called my neighbor and a friend and asked them to come to my home to stay with me. When your husband called to tell me of your mastectomy, I broke down and was not able to talk to him. That night, after you had come out of the anesthetic, you called me, and talking to you helped calm my anxiety.

I visited you as soon as I could and was with you when your doctor called to tell you about needing six months of chemotherapy. I thought you were brave about it even though you cried as we sat there holding hands.

You withstood the chemo well, even though you were very weak and tired and had to buy a wig because you were losing your hair. Your father lost his hair three times. You seemed to get very depressed and wondered what was going to happen to you.

As time went on, you improved and looked much better. You were acting more normal. I believe being able to go back to your school work and church activities, the love of your many friends and relatives, especially your husband, sons, sister and me, made it all seem easier to take.

As a mother, when one of your children hurt, you suffer with them."

From my one and only sister, six years my elder:

"Free association of my reaction—

1) fear and grief: Your husband called me at work. He was crying. I was crying. I worried about Mom and wanted to set up support for her.

2) at hospital: I felt empathy about losing a breast. I identified with that for weeks and wondered how it would be. I admired your spirit, strength, and sense of humor.

3) worried you might die: I would lose you as a friend and support person. I thought about how important you are to Mom. You would not be here to face old age with me and to help with Mom and our other relatives. I would be all alone.

4) anger about your prior depression,
   which I felt led to depressed immune
   system and, thus, cancer.

5) worried you might hate me because
   I'm older and should have major illness
   first. It's not fair.

6) worried about my daughters and
   wondered if this will pass to them.

7) glad that people in your community
   were supportive and validated your
   contribution to them."

From my aunt, my father's sister:

"I'm afraid I am a very poor subject to respond to your questions. I've never been one to be able to put my deepest emotions into words. I've always had a deep-seated aversion to talking about something that possibly could happen or something I truly wanted to happen. It is as though talking about it and dwelling on it will cause the reverse to happen.

I always thought that I was the only one in my family that felt that way until you happened to mention that you didn't know how your Dad managed all those years without dwelling on or talking about the cancer he had in the 1940's. It made me realize that he must have had the same aversion.

When I first heard about your problem, I was sad that one of my favorite people had to face this trauma; then, I started thinking of all the women I knew who had gone through the same thing. Among them were two close friends who had the operation about thirty years ago and haven't slowed down since.

Knowing the advances that have been made in the medical field over the past years, I was confident that, although you would have a long period of pain and discomfort to face, you would be able to handle it with your usual determination and your chin out.

The one time I really panicked was the day of your operation. Your mother told me she would call to give us the outcome as soon as she heard. When it got to be eleven o'clock that night, and I still hadn't heard, I was very concerned and called your sister.

As to how we view you after this shattering experience, to us you are the same loved niece you always were. We always were very proud of your achievements and this is no exception."

From my college roommate and longtime friend:

"CANCER: the big 'C'.

HOPE: When the initial surgery was scheduled, hope filled my mind and there was no doubt but that the surgery would be minor and the tumor benign. Throughout our years of friendship, our 'group' had seemingly been immune to any major illnesses or problems.

This fairy-tale existence was about to continue.

DENIAL: Calling to supposedly hear the good news brought a message of despair. This couldn't be happening—I must have heard wrong—the doctor made a mistake. If I don't think about it, it will have just been a bad dream.

QUESTIONING: Why my friend? Why not me? What is she feeling now? What thoughts does she have?

EMPATHY: Questioning and concern gave way to such strong feelings of empathy that I became, in my mind, my friend. I had pain. I tried to foresee my future and how I would deal with the diagnosis.

FRUSTRATION: Wanting so badly to be of help, to make everything whole and well again. I wanted to be in close proximity, needing to be in her company more.

HOPE: Visiting at the hospital made me aware of my friend's strength in coping, of her ability to be in control of her life, now, as she always has been. She was dealing with the situation much better than I.

QUESTIONING: Another period of questioning began and lasted for the six months of chemotherapy. Was this truly necessary? The weakness and loss of energy were almost too much to watch in a person who has always had so much drive.

We continue together in the seemingly circle of hope, unanswered questions and frustrations. We have become closer, enjoying time spent together reminiscing. Each day becomes more precious. We realize that we aren't infinite beings.

My friend's illness has made me more daring, willing to take more risks. I want to do things now and not put them off. Together we plan a 'dream vacation' to celebrate life and God's love and grace to all of u s."

[Note: Two of my college roommates and our spouses traveled to Hawaii for a ten-day vacation. We definitely pushed the "edge" when we crossed over a barrier and walked on crusted lava with cracks showing flowing lava beneath our feet.]

From my niece: (written in the third person)

" 'Oh, no!' said the girl. It had been a normal day, just like any other, until now. She had just heard that her aunt has breast cancer and is undergoing surgery that will remove one of her breasts. Her breasts! She is still so young.

Is there a possibility that the cancer has spread to other parts of her body? Death! The thoughts flew wildly through the girl's head.

She had been concerned about her aunt for several years now. She was not just any relative. This aunt was special, her mother's only sister.

She had known her aunt all her life. As a little girl she had gone to her aunt's wedding, and she could still remember their youthful faces.

They had watched the changes through each other's lives. She had gone on vacation with their family to Washington, D.C. This aunt had shared the loss of the girl's father.

Cancer—that dirty word. Could this have been the stimulus for her aunt's recent period of depression, those hollow cheeks and the increasing loss of weight?

Cancer! She must be afraid. She has worked so hard all her life, and now this. The girl felt so awful and afraid for her.

She hoped the operation and the following chemotherapy treatments would be successful and not too much for her already weakened spirit and body.

The operation—her breasts! Breasts seem to mean so much to the identity of a woman. It's irrational. At the thought of losing them, the girl suddenly feels glad for what she has, even though they are small. How stupid. Our bodies. Why must we be so obsessed with our bodies?

Death—no, she is too young. This would be so awful, so unfair. The girl refused to acknowledge this possibility, but the worry persisted.

Time passes. The girl lives so far away from the ongoing trauma, yet, thinks of her aunt between her busy hours. She sends some flowers and a card. She waits for news from her mother.

The chemotherapy begins. The strength of her aunt impresses the girl. She worries about her uncle's ability to adjust. Our bodies. Why always our bodies? She is losing her hair. The chemotherapy weakens her; yet, she paints a room in her house.

Time passes. She is getting better. The girl sees her aunt over the holidays. The hollowness is leaving her face. She seems to be gaining weight. The girl feels relief.

The cycle closes for the girl, but she knows that it will remain with her aunt. She is glad to hear that her aunt has begun an exercise program. It will be good for her body. Our bodies are important. It will ease her mind."

From my youngest niece:

"I believe that I am a person not easily shocked by bad news. My personal experience with disaster (accident and death of my father), and my work as a physical therapist with people who have experienced disasters (quadriplegia, stroke, Multiple Sclerosis, etc.) has given me a more realistic or harder view of illness and death.

After hearing about your previous breast cysts and knowing about your recent episode of depression, I was not shocked with the news that you had cancer and would need a modified radical mastectomy. I was very much saddened that you would have to deal with yet another personal hardship!

I believe I called you soon after I heard the news and offered some support. I was scared to call because I didn't know what to say. Even though I deal with people who have suffered with many different diseases and problems in the hospital setting, this situation was one I had to deal with directly on a more personal level.

I would not call myself a 'huggy' person and always have to convince myself to give a hug or offer verbal support in a difficult situation. This is an area that I constantly work

on since I know how much better I feel when others hug me and offer me comforting thoughts. I wish I had been able to do more for you!

Knowing that you had to have a modified radical mastectomy, I wondered how it would affect your image of yourself. I know several other women who have lost one or both breasts and appear to be functioning normally; physically and psychologically. I have not been close enough to any of these women to really help them deal with these changes in their bodies.

Looking at the psychological aspect of dealing with a medical problem such as cancer, I was concerned that you were burying yourself in so much work and activity that you didn't have time to actually face the issue.

Kubler-Ross, who wrote on this topic might call this time period denial, since it seemed you acted like nothing was wrong and didn't realize that your mind and body needed

rest. I am glad that you have finally cut back on work and are involved in regular physical exercise. I believe that regular exercise is not only physically stimulating but psychologically uplifting as well.

The fear of cancer seems to follow us wherever we go. We constantly hear speculation on causes and very little on cure. Over Christmas I had my first taste of that fear for myself. When I developed abnormally swollen glands throughout my body, I immediately thought of Hodgkin's Disease. Well, I let the doctor know my fears and was thankful to find out it was only an allergy to sulfa medication. This experience made me realize how vulnerable we all are to the fear of the unknown."

From the friend who was in prison:

"As I reflect back on a year ago, I recall your first letter informing me of your surgery and pending recuperation. My first remembrance was that I said to myself, 'Oh my God, what else does she have to face? Enough is enough. Why her?'

I then felt a closer kinship with you as I related it to my situation; indeed, I've faced a different cancer - less externally obvious but nonetheless real. It, too, had to be treated before wellness was possible. If not treated, it might have also spread.

At that time, I had been in therapy for close to a year and had passed through much self-searching. I related to your experiences through mine, translated into physical and spiritual terms and felt empathy. I hope that has shown through in my letters to you.

I think the thing that touched me most deeply might be considered a small thing. You shared the card (drawing) you did of the daffodils and then asked me to return it to you after a while. It was like having a great masterpiece on display at my home, on loan. It meant much to me because I knew how much effort it took to accomplish this visual expression.

I felt over the long haul we both grew to a deeper understanding of each other, as fellow human beings along life's road. You have shared inner feelings with me as I have with you.

For me it only can enhance my appreciation of your victories because I have been privileged to walk with you through the battles and near defeats. Your struggles have helped me in part face my own inadequacies and added some strength to my endeavors. I feel quite comfortable being called a friend along life's way."

MY RESPONSE – 1988

"There is no adequate way to say thank you to you, my family and friends. As I look at each response, I am aware of the effort required to answer my questions. I am impressed with the thoughtfulness given to this task.

When I received and read each letter, there was an overwhelming sense of love and strength that radiated into the depths of my being.

Thank you."

When I read through the responses as a collection, I was fascinated with the overlapping and interweaving of themes. They coincided to a great degree with many of the feelings that I expressed in poetry at the age of 46. The support that is so evident carried me into the next phase of my unknown journey with even greater strength.

While recuperating from the mastectomy, my oldest son was diagnosed with mononucleosis and wanted to come home. He took one sofa, and I took the other. We didn't talk about cancer, and that was okay.

My youngest son was a high school senior, busy with school activities. One evening after I was told I would need chemotherapy, I was in a daze.

There was a half-finished puzzle on the dining room table, and I sat down to work on it. He joined me. That was when I told him about the need for chemotherapy and I didn't intend to die of cancer. His response was that "I would probably get hit by a car on the way to my doctor's office for my last IV." That's my boy!

Depression began several years prior to the diagnosis of breast cancer and continued

to be a major problem, and even though I was taking medication, the inability to work, coupled with the gray days of Ohio, took their toll. I sought counseling from my pastor, and he led me down a destructive path in order to satisfy his needs, adding more stress to my life.

My first marriage wasn't strong enough to endure and ended in divorce. Ultimately, years of professional therapy helped me get back on my feet.

One day as I waited in my car for a traffic light to turn from red to green, I watched a squirrel on a telephone wire that went across the street high above my head. The tiny gray squirrel scampered a third of the way across and lost his balance. I watched curiously as he righted himself and continued on.

Suddenly he toppled again, yet held on to the wire and righted himself once more. I hoped traffic would not force me to move on before this drama was complete.

Would you believe this squirrel lost his balance again? This time I laughed and was amazed to see it complete the journey upside down on that flimsy wire. I realized that, in that position, one can only look up.

My life since 1987 has been much like that of the squirrel. While I survived the cancer, the treatment caused ongoing problems. We don't know why, but chemotherapy substantially weakened my legs and no amount of exercise has brought them back to normal.

After my physical and emotional strength improved, I accepted a position in a school district 25 miles from home.

This job as an elementary school counselor required me to be up and down the staircase numerous times a day. Sometimes I stood at the bottom, looking up, not sure I had the strength to go to the third floor where my office was located.

When I couldn't hear the children's voices, evaluation showed hearing loss in the middle ear. The tiny bones had calcified, probably from chemotherapy. This was corrected by surgery to place a tiny wire through the bone and it worked.

There were days when I would be tired after driving to work. My patience was not what it used to be. I would make a phone call and repeat it a half hour later, with no recall. The problems of the children and their families overwhelmed me. Ultimately, I was placed on disability retirement.

A GENERATION LATER

My mother, aunt, first husband, and my sister have passed on. My nieces live in Sequim, Washington and Williamsburg, Virginia; about as far from each other as you can get and also far from me in Arizona.

I will always be grateful that my nieces arranged a week vacation for the two of them, plus my sister and me. That was in April of 2015 and my sister died suddenly in November.

My oldest son is married and has an adult son. My youngest son is married and has a teenager. They live in Ohio and I live in Arizona. My college friends are busy with their families. We see each other when possible.

Although cancer is everywhere, I don't think about it much anymore. A mammogram can raise my heartbeat and has always been a blip on my radar.

I married Charles Barnhart in 1992. He had been my masseur for three years. Following divorce from my first husband, we began to date. He taught me to say, "I love you." That had been lacking in my life to that point. Now, my sons and their families speak of love with their wives and children. My heart swells. Charlie never fails to express his love to his daughter, three grandchildren, and the great-grandchildren. And now, I have learned to do the same.

Charlie is totally blind and has been since he was ten years old. A virus destroyed his optic nerve. Even so, he is quite independent. From ages 10 to 17 he lived and studied at the School for the Blind in Columbus, Ohio. I also lived in Columbus for the first 25 years of my life.

I find it quite amusing that we married. When I was a freshman in college, I dated a guy who had been blind since birth. After our third date my mother asked, "You aren't going to marry a blind man are you?" What did I do? I married a blind man.

Mom adjusted, and one time when she was visiting, she asked Charlie for a massage! My mother really did that. She also learned to say, "I love you."

Following the birth of my oldest son, I became restless staying home. After three months I put my name in as a substitute teacher.

One of my assignments sent me to a classroom for five months. I encountered a fourth grade girl who had been blind since birth. She had Braille textbooks, a Braille writer and typewriter at her desk. I had no training or experience teaching a student who was blind.

My lesson plans for physical education included volleyball. I was concerned about my blind student's safety and asked her to help me keep score. She walked out of the gym and went home to her mother. She wanted to play volleyball, and her mother walked back to school with her and said it was OK. She taught me not to assume, and to ask her how she would handle any given activity.

My last job before going on disability was in Springfield, Ohio. I learned even more from a teacher who was blind. She taught a class for the blind and visually impaired and helped me understand that blindness limits a person in some ways but not in all ways. There are other ways of seeing. She had a guide dog, owned her own home, and had an assistant in her third floor classroom. She took either a city bus or cab to school.

We became friends and ate out together frequently. After two unpleasant surprises, she asked me to please let her know when she encountered something on her plate that she couldn't see, such as the anchovy in a Greek salad or a blob of butter on the pancakes.

When it became evident that I was not able to continue working, I was placed on Disability Retirement. My cancer treatment in 1987 prevented me from remaining in my career. Body weakness keeps bringing me back to a reality I still have difficulty accepting.

Living in Tucson has worked well for Charlie and me. He has door-to-door transportation and activities for the visually impaired at Southern Arizona Association for the Blind. One day he makes greeting cards and on another he sands and cleans pottery before painting glaze on it. His teacher comes up with clever ideas on the third day he is there.

At home he makes the bed, does the laundry (after I sort it), manages the dishwasher, takes the garbage out, and any other household chore I can think of. He even talked our mail carrier into putting a rubber band around our mail so when he takes it out of the box he won't drop anything.

We exercise three days a week and attend activities at church as well as worship on Sundays,

Some days we go to movies. Every movie theater is required to offer a head set and transistor which provides the blind with audio description. This allows the patron to know all of the non-verbal things that are going on. We have season passes to our local theater that also provides description. Then too, Charlie would be lost without books to listen to along with his SiriusXM radio.

One of our favorite places to go is atop Mt. Lemmon. It takes an hour to make the drive up where we enjoy a big cookie or some other goodie. The temperature is twenty degrees cooler and is a relief from the summer heat.

I have been trained and commissioned as a Stephen Minister for our church. In addition to meetings twice a month, we are assigned to a person experiencing difficult times, and walk along their path with them. Looking to God as we meet, we bring prayer, Scripture, and listening ears.

THE DAFFODIL STORY

The day I was discharged from the hospital, I took with me a bouquet of daffodils. To me, they were a symbol that I had cancer because they had been purchased from a fund-raiser of our local American Cancer Society. I carried them stoically even though I did not want them.

In my mind I thought about dropping them in a wastebasket as my wheelchair went down the hall. However that was out of character for me so I took them home.

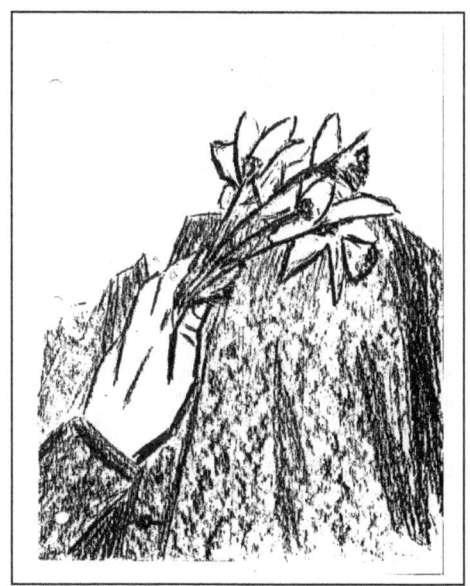

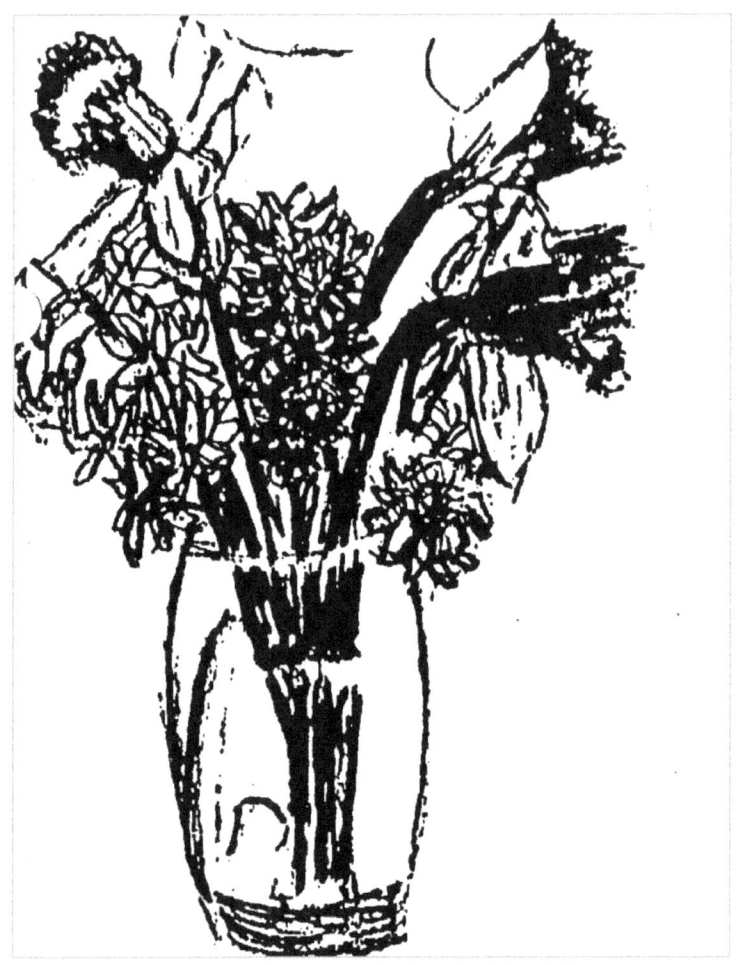

Easter arrived and someone gave me a bouquet of
daffodils and hyacinths. They were beautiful
sitting on my kitchen table, especially when the sun
shone on them. However, within two weeks they
died.

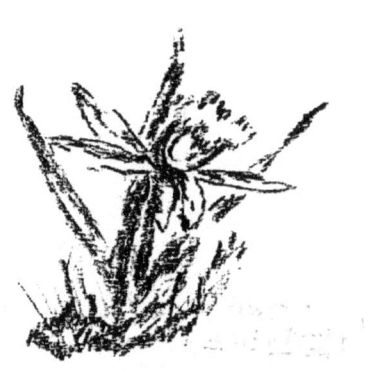

The day I saw
daffodils growing in
a neighbor's garden,
I immediately knew
these were the
flowers with the
most meaning. These
daffodils were
rooted in the earth.
Although they would
die, they would rise
again in a year.

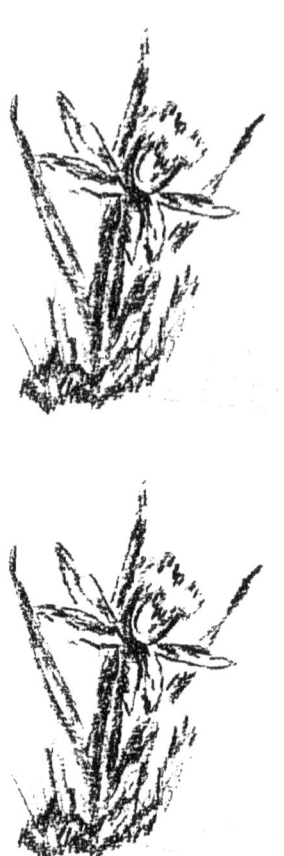

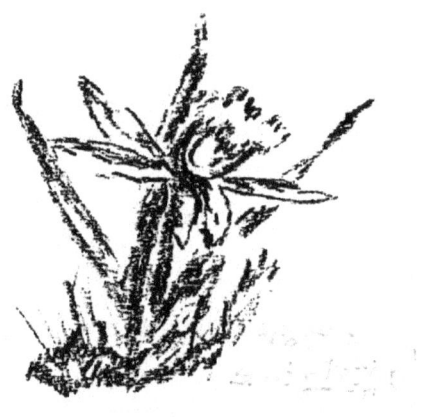

RESTING IN THE ARMS OF MY CREATOR

I rest in the arms of God, the Creator, who brought order out of chaos. God reigns—robed in majesty, girded with strength. He is mightier than the waves of the sea, yet, gentle enough to cradle a baby.

I believe God placed his Son on this earth so all could learn from his example. God sacrificed His Son for me, just as the prophets foretold.

I believe God, the Holy Spirit, intervenes in my mind, gives me ideas, and helps me make decisions. He leads others into my path and leads me into the paths of others. He shows me his love and the way of peace.

I view my life as a stage, a span. And I view death as a transition to another existence that God, in infinite wisdom, has also designed.

"I WAS THERE TO HEAR YOUR BORNING CRY"

~~John Ylvisaker

I was there to hear your borning cry,
I'll be there when you are old.
I rejoiced the day you were baptized,
to see your life unfold.

I was there when you were but a child,
with a faith to suit you well;
in a blaze of light you wandered off
to find where demons dwell.

When you heard the wonder of the Word
I was there to cheer you on;
you were raised to praise the living Lord,
to whom you now belong.

If you find someone to share your time
and you join your hearts as one,
I'll be there to make your verses rhyme
from dusk till rising sun.

Breast Cancer, an Emotional Journey

In the middle ages of your life,
not too old, no longer young,
I'll be there to guide you through the night,
complete what I've begun.

When the evening gently closes in
and you shut your weary eyes,
I'll be there as I have always been
with just one more surprise.

I was there to hear your borning cry,
I'll be there when you are old.
I rejoiced the day you were baptized,
to see your life unfold.

Thank you for reading about my breast cancer experience. I hope you will share the story with others who have the same or similar diagnoses, or their family and friends.

I have also authored and published "PERSONAL ENCOUNTERS WITH CANCER" [lung, prostate, breast metastases, bladder, tongue and breast] These are stories of six different people with six different kinds of cancer.

Both books are available through Amazon and Kindle. You can download a Kindle app for tablets and other readers. Bookstores around the world will order the book for you through (Print on Demand).

Check my author website for information about speaking engagements.

www.margaretbarnhart.com

www.ingramcontent.com/pod-product-compliance
Lightning Source LLC
Chambersburg PA
CBHW070147290526
45789CB00002B/660